The Power of Positivity

The Power of Positivity

Eighty ways to energize your life

Joel and Ruth Schroeder

SkillPath Publications

Mission, KS

Project Editor: Kelly Scanlon

Editor: Jane Doyle Guthrie

Page Layout: Premila Malik Borchardt

Cover Design: Rod Hankins

ISBN: 1-57294-068-9

Library of Congress Catalog Card Number: 96-69969

10 9 8 7 6 5 4 3 2 1   02 03 04 05

Printed in the United States of America

Contents

Introduction 1

1. Puttin' on the Ritz 3

2. Back to Nature 4

3. Open Your Mind's Eye 5

4. Stop! 7

5. Don't Start at the Beginning 9

6. Rewrite History 10

7. Hidden Purple Power 11

8. The Joy Touch 12

9. Write On 13

10. The Power of Example 14

11. Listen to the Beat 15

12. "X" Marks the Spot 16

13. No Double Standards 17

14. Look on the Bright Side 18

15. A Change of Venue 19

16. Rest on Your Laurels 20

17. Don't Sweat It . . . Sweat! 21

18. Count Your Blessings 22

19. Come to Your Senses 23

20. Change Your Focus 25

21. Say "Cheese" 26

22. Declare a Grieving Period 27

23. Wash Away Your Troubles 28

24. Game Time 29

25. "Lucky" Pennies 30

26. Grab Your Eyebrows 31

27. Add to Your Joy List 32

28. Candy Is Dandy 33

29. Silent Scream 34

30. What's So Funny About This? 35

31. Reframe It 36

32. Early to Bed 37

33. Take a Deep Breath 38

34. Toys Aren't Just for Kids 39

35. Affirm It 40

36. Rx: See Your Doctor 42

37. Make It Worse 43

38. Dial-a-Smile 44

39. It's Contagious 45

40. Use Your Mental Earplugs 46

41. Do the Can-Can 47

42. Ask the Right Questions 48

43. Get Spiritual 49

44. Say "Ouch" 50

45. Up Your Stroke/Poke Ratio 51

46. Hang It Up 52

47. Don't Should on Yourself or Others 53

48. Ain't It a Shame! 54

49. Be Agreeable 55

50. Trace Your Roots 56

51. Change Your Hat 57

52. Eyes on the Prize 58

53. Sounding Boards 59

54. This Is Dedicated to the One I Love 60

55. Put a Price Tag on It 61

56. Shifting Gears 62

57. 3:2:1 63

58. Step by Step 64

59. Tape Your Negativity Shut 65

60. Try a Little Tenderness 67

61. Under the Dumping Tree 68

62. Extending a Helping Hand 69

63. Come to Your Senses 70

64. Learn Something New 71

65. Philosophy of Positivity 72

66. Take Over the Controls 73

67. Testing 1… 2… 3 74

68. Do Your Dirty Work 75

69. Back to the Future 76

70. Time Out 77

71. Go, Team, Go! 78

72. Quitting Time 79

73. Climb to Common Ground 80

74. A Word From the Wise 81

75. Do Nothing 82

76. Reward Yourself 83

77. Script It 84

78. Danger! Keep Out!! 85

79. Whine Country 86

80. Rela-a-a-x 87

Bibliography and Suggested Reading 89

Introduction

Zig Ziglar was right—your *attitude* does determine your *altitude.*

- Take injured gymnast Kerri Strug. She vaulted to 1996 Olympic gold and into America's heart while telling herself, "I will do it! I will, I will, I will!"

- Attitudes can affect your health. Studies show that grieving spouses have weakened immune systems. They have fewer T-cells, the kind of white blood cells that attack harmful invaders into their bodies.

- Orville Redenbacher kept believing he had created a superior brand of popcorn. Farmers, wholesalers, and retailers told him the public wouldn't pay a premium for gourmet popcorn. Positive-thinking Redenbacher's higher-priced popcorn still rules the Kingdom of Popcorn.

Success. Health. Wealth. A positive attitude plays a leading role in each.

But attitudes are contagious—bad ones as well as good ones. We are faced with negative situations, irritating people, and tiresome tasks. Faced with these, emotional batteries run down. So we need all the tools we can find to bring a positive charge to our attitude and lives.

Here are 80 ways to do that. Eighty ways to power a spirit soaring in the stratosphere. Or 80 ways to power the liftoff of a body glued below sea level by what feels like 3 G's of emotional gravity.

1

Puttin' on the Ritz

You're someone special, and when you dress that way, you'll feel that way. Deck out in your best duds and head for a fabulous restaurant or tony event with someone who also gets into the spirit of "dress up." Go out and sparkle for a couple of hours.

"Only those who dare to fail miserably can achieve greatly." Robert F. Kennedy

2

Back to Nature

When you need to retreat from pressure and negativity, contact with Nature can leave you refreshed and recharged. Is it the beauty of the lake or woods that does it? The awesome majesty of the ocean or mountains? The quiet? The colors and fragrances? The randomness embraced in a sense of eternal order? Or is it just being away from phones, faxes, and forms?

Getting back to nature doesn't have to mean an hour-long drive to a state park, though. Make the day's troubles fade by stepping onto your back porch and using sunflower seeds to coax the cardinals a little closer in. Or during the day, spend five minutes away from your hermetically sealed, temperature-controlled office and just let the breeze blow across your skin.

"Believe that life is worth living, and your belief will help create the fact." William James

3

Open Your Mind's Eye

A prisoner of war endured unspeakable tortures by playing a four-hour round of golf every day in his mind. He hit perfectly, shot after shot; he saw and heard the birds, smelled the grass, impatiently waited for slow foursomes putzing around on the green ahead of his group.

The result? In his first round of golf after he was released, he shot in the low 70s—an improvement of 20 strokes below his average round before his capture.

You're not a prisoner of war, but sometimes you *do* feel trapped, helpless, and hopeless. Do what the other prisoners did—control *one* place in the universe, your mind.

Mental diversions and visualization not only distract you from present difficulties, the process fires the same neurons you use when you actually perform the activity you're visualizing. You could plan your next weekend getaway, mentally overhaul your '69 Corvette's engine, or run around the track at the nearby college campus.

Tap regularly into these vast mental resources you've probably never explored, and see how your performance improves as well as your mood.

"To believe a thing is impossible is to make it so." French proverb

Stop!

If you are prone to talk to yourself negatively ("That was really stupid!"), stop it!

Hold out your hand like a cop directing traffic and say firmly, "Stop!" The command will go deeper into your consciousness if your ears actually hear that word said in that way.

However, you may rightly fear that if you bark this order where others can hear, they might come after you with a butterfly net. So if others are present, *write* "Stop," or *visualize* a red stop sign.

Jack Canfield suggests a similar technique in his cassette tape series *How to Build High Self-Esteem.* Canfield suggests saying "Cancel, cancel" after you've said negative things to yourself (or if others speak that way to you). After doing this, add a positive statement that contradicts the negative message, perhaps like this: "Cancel, cancel—I am an intelligent human being," or "Cancel, cancel—no matter what you say or do to me, I'm still a worthwhile person."

"No man knows what he can do till he tries." Publilius Syrus

5

Don't Start at the Beginning

Get in the habit of focusing on the desired *result* at the beginning of the challenge. With an eye on what you want, hope, and expect to be, you can endure the bumps, bruises, and lumps it takes to get there more easily.

And real power comes from anticipating the feelings you'll have at the end. Can you picture how you'll enjoy the "attaboys" or "attagirls"? Can you see the smiles of appreciation and admiration? Can you already touch that finished report or fine furniture you've crafted? Can you smell that first loaf of homemade bread? Yes, you can.

And tapping into those feelings now will help make those results come true.

> "There is nothing like a dream to create the future." Victor Hugo

6

Rewrite History

When you're feeling like the world's worst failure, put a new shine on your résumé. If you were interviewing for a once-in-a-lifetime job tomorrow, what good things would you want to say about yourself? Have you won an award? Attended some professional or self-improvement seminars? If you were describing someone else with your skills and background, what accomplishments would you feature?

Chances are, you'll end up feeling pretty impressed. And if you don't stay in your corner, who will?

"If your ship doesn't come in, swim out to it." Jonathan Winters

Hidden Purple Power

A successful woman once revealed, "When I face an extremely challenging day, I wear my matching purple underwear. Nobody else knows my secret. But I know when I wear these things, you'd better not mess with me. I can't be stopped!"

If lavender lingerie doesn't fit your power fantasy, imagine wearing a bulletproof vest. You are invincible!

"He that respects himself is safe from others; he wears a coat of mail that none can pierce." Henry Wadsworth Longfellow

8

The Joy Touch

Pete Sanders of Sedona, Arizona, describes a simple biofeedback technique he calls the "Joy Touch."

Picture a line running from the center of your forehead to the center of your brain. This is the site of the *septum pellucidum,* a sort of remote control for the pleasure center of your brain.

Focus your thoughts as high as your eyes, then higher. Think about gently brushing or stroking that part of your brain, just as you'd pet your dog or your cat.

For some users, this technique is a three-second autobahn to the alpha state, relieving their stress and controlling their heartbeat.

"Gray skies are just clouds passing over."
Duke Ellington

9

Write On

Why do counselors recommend journaling? Because by writing your thoughts, you figuratively dump them out on the table, where you can see what's happening more objectively.

Did you know that people who journal after losing their jobs in a downsizing get new jobs faster? They deal with their fears, anger, and hurt on paper. They lay plans and articulate clear strategies. Journaling helps us deal with our emotions constructively in private, not in the heat of battle.

"Never let fear intrude on what you know."
Sun Rain, American Indian philosopher

10

The Power of Example

Treat yourself to reading a biography or autobiography when you feel shaky or uncertain. In almost every case, you'll see ways the subject overcame adversity before becoming rich, successful, famous, or whatever the claim to fame. It's never easy. It wasn't for them, and it won't be for you. But the fortification of their examples will inspire you to face down your dragons, to navigate the hurdles that seem too tall or wide to get around.

Remember, the road to mediocrity is straight and smooth—because it's well worn.

"I've never seen a monument erected to a pessimist." Paul Harvey

11

Listen to the Beat

Music has power, and not just to soothe the savage breast. It motivates and inspires. The "Battle Hymn of the Republic" and "Dixie" helped the Union and Confederate armies keep going through death, deprivation, and despair. College teams have "fight songs," and the Seven Dwarves all whistled while they worked.

What notes inspire you? Whether stirring or calming, choose music that makes you feel good, alive, positive, and hopeful. Put together a tape of the special inspirational favorites that never fail to juice your attitude.

"One can never consent to creep when one feels an impulse to soar." Helen Keller

12

"X" Marks the Spot

Think of one of your happiest moments. How did you feel? Relive the emotions as vividly as you can.

Now touch any spot on your body—just above your watch, or on your forearm, or somewhere else that is easily reached and unobtrusive. This spot will be your trigger. Touch the spot and relive the emotions of that happiest moment. Repeat until you've programmed your emotions to respond with joy when you touch that spot.

You can set similar triggers to revisit and repeat peak performances, when you were "at the top of your game." Touch the spot you've programmed and feel the emotions. They can help harness those thoughts and skills that bring you back to the level of success you've patterned.

Scientists call this NLP—neurolinguistic programming. Call it what you will. It works!

"You will draw to yourself that which you most persistently think about." Anonymous

13

No Double Standards

How would your situation look to you if it were someone else in the picture? What would you say to a friend going through a similar experience? If he'd just been through a tough job interview, could you imagine scolding him with "Why weren't you better prepared? You really blew it! You'll probably never get a job now"?

No, of course not. You'd reassure him and say, "You'll find another good job. That was their mistake not to hire you." So don't use a double standard. Talk to yourself with the same kindness and understanding you'd show your best friend.

> "People often say that this or that person has not yet found himself. But the self is not something that one finds. It is something that one creates." Thomas Szasz

14

Look on the Bright Side

In the midst of a shower of negativity, brainstorm. What good can come out of this? Can you learn anything about yourself or others? Will it lead to more patience or empathy for others? Will this be a hard-earned lesson you can pass on so others won't experience it?

Even ridiculous thoughts help. "Well . . . at least this will keep me from becoming so famous that all the skeletons in my closet will be discovered."

"Our greatest glory is not in never falling but in rising every time we fall." Confucius

15

A Change of Venue

Don't just sit there. Go somewhere. Walk. Run. Ride. A change of scenery can do wonders for your outlook. Even leaving the building for lunch can give you a whole new perspective.

Walking or running has the added benefit of doing something constructive with the adrenaline pumping into your bloodstream because of the flight-fight response. You don't want to fight. So flee, already!

And if you can't go somewhere literally, *travel in your mind* to a favorite refuge, to a quiet, delightful place where you feel at peace. Circumstances may prevent you from going there in a car or plane, but nothing can keep you from an imaginary visit.

"Work is the greatest thing in the world, so we should always save some of it for tomorrow." Don Herold

16

Rest on Your Laurels

When someone compliments you, notice and enjoy it instead of just shrugging it off with an uncomfortable "Oh, it was nothing," or a quick little "Thank you."

But that's not all. Start a compliment file, sort of like saving pennies for a rainy day. Record every compliment you receive, listing who said it and what prompted the kind words.

When you're feeling down or unappreciated, open your compliment "piggy bank" and read what nice things folks have said about you. Now trust their good judgment.

"No one can make you feel inferior without your consent." Eleanor Roosevelt

17

Don't Sweat It . . . Sweat!

Channel the energy that's keeping you stirred up and seething into calisthenics or aerobics. Lift weights—pound the treadmill—use the stair climber as a ladder out of your funk!

Exercise helps exhaust immediate stress, and it will train your heart and circulatory system to handle future bouts more effectively.

"Not failure, but low aim, is a crime."
James Russell Lowell

18

Count Your Blessings

Maybe you've had a rough day, week, month, year, or even decade. (Life, anyone?) Is there *anything* still going well for you? What *can* you still be thankful for? Your health? Family? Partner? Kids? Friends? Job? Church? Maybe your naturally curly hair?

The more you look for blessings, and the more blessings you find to appreciate, the smaller your present challenges will look by comparison.

"We are too soon old, and too late smart."
Hebrew Proverb

19

Come to Your Senses

Our sense of smell is more powerful than most of us imagine. We can distinguish 10,000 distinct smells. Babies can recognize their mothers by smell alone.

While all the senses can trigger good or bad memories, some researchers indicate that the sense of smell may be the quickest way. Scents stimulate the limbic system, where feelings and long-term memory reside. The smell of pumpkin pie or fresh pine may flood you with memories of happy celebrations at Thanksgiving and Christmas. Bacon and eggs frying may evoke positive scenes of a late-morning breakfast in the cottage on the lake you visited as a child. Peanut butter cookies might call to mind Grandma's round kitchen table with its vinyl checkerboard tablecloth.

Most Americans (culture matters in aromatherapy) react to the following smells in predictable ways:

Vanilla	Relieves depression
Peppermint, rosemary, lemon, juniper, and eucalyptus	Enhance concentration, lift mood, improve productivity
Jasmine, basil	Stimulate
Sandalwood, musk, cinnamon	Stir sensual response

Lavender	Reduces brain wave activity, relaxes
Nutmeg, cedar, fir	Lowers blood pressure

So how can you use your knowledge of these aromas or essences? A bubble bath is one way. A hot compress with a washcloth also can be very refreshing. Put the scent into boiling water and breathe the mixture deeply with a towel draped over your head. Dab a few drops of fragrance on a lamp's wire frame. The heat will dispense the fragrance. A Japanese company saw productivity increase when they pumped lemon aroma through the air conditioner.

You can also train your body to associate a particular smell with a particular mood. Always use a vanilla essence in a relaxing bath. After half a dozen times, the smell of vanilla will relax you—without the bath!

"Opportunity does not come to those who wait. It is captured by those who attack."
General Douglas MacArthur

20

Change Your Focus

The more you focus on yourself during serious problems, the worse they seem to look, and grow. Change your focus! Turn your view finder optimistically toward others.

John F. Kennedy said, "Ask not what your country can do for you; ask what you can do for your country," and Americans canonized him. Jimmy Carter told voters the country was in a malaise and citizens would have to suffer; they picked another leader at the polls. In fact, Americans elected the more optimistic candidate for president eighteen out of twenty-two times from 1900 to 1988.

Focusing outward optimistically works for average folks too—not just presidential hopefuls!

"Men are not prisoners of fate, but only prisoners of their own minds." Franklin D. Roosevelt

21

Say "Cheese"

"If you have any troubles, they will vanish like a bubble, if you only take the trouble just to S-M-I-L-E."

Remember that silly song? The truth it expresses isn't so silly after all. It's almost impossible to give a smile away—the instant you send it toward another person, you'll see it coming back again. Boomerang style, it knocks out your tension and makes you feel better.

And because it takes forty-three muscles to frown but only seventeen to smile, it saves all that wear and tear on your face.

"He who waits for a roast duck to fly in his mouth must wait a very, very long time."
Chinese proverb

22

Declare a Grieving Period

You missed the promotion you were hoping for. You passed a major birthday milestone that spells goodbye to your youth. You had a camping trip planned, but now you have to work all weekend instead.

Often depression follows a loss we haven't clearly identified as such. When you recognize a loss, declare a fixed time to grieve over it.

Instead of enduring an unproductive and prolonged period of undefined sadness, give yourself permission to mourn or feel disappointed. Tell yourself how long you expect it to last, and actually clock yourself if need be. Do special things for yourself during this time, and generally cut yourself a little slack!

When your declared grieving time is over, see if you don't feel ready to tackle "normal" life again.

"A woman is like a teabag; you never know how strong she is until she gets in hot water." Nancy Reagan

23

Wash Away Your Troubles

You're upset. The adrenaline is pumping through your body, preparing you to spring into action.

Why not kill two birds with one stone? Use your stress-induced energy to eliminate another downer—how about your cluttered basement or sticky-to-the-step kitchen floor?

When the floor is clean enough to eat off of, your attitude will be a lot brighter too. And as you're sorting Christmas ornaments and garden tools onto shelves downstairs, the repetition will throw your thoughts onto the right side of your brain—the side of play and creative thinking.

That's a fun place to be, and spending time there will help give you a different perspective on your troubles. Maybe even turn up a creative solution or two.

"They who lose today may win tomorrow."
Michael Cervantes

Game Time

Do you remember how your mom, dad, or teachers made work seem fun when they turned it into a game? Take the unpleasant task or duty facing you and do the same thing:

- Can I type this report in an hour and make fewer than two errors per page?

- Can I finish straightening the house before my partner returns from the grocery store?

- Can I write at least one page every day?

- Can I dress up this proposal with graphics to give it a professional layout?

- Can I balance these accounts on my first try?

- Can I relocate this dock full of barrels in two hours?

Play your way through that job you are dreading.

"The wise don't expect to find life worth living; they make it that way." Anonymous

25

"Lucky" Pennies

A mother told her children it was lucky to find a "heads up" penny.

Guess what she regularly hid around her home, especially when the kids were experiencing difficulties? When her sons and daughters, disgruntled over something, ran across a penny, they immediately stopped to look. When it was "heads up," their frowns always changed to smiles.

"A diamond is a chunk of coal that made good under pressure." Anonymous

Grab Your Eyebrows

Feeling tense? Touch your eyebrows. They'll quickly tell your fingertips just how much stress you're under. You'll *feel* how your face *looks* to others.

Push your eyebrows toward your ears with your thumb or index finger. You'll feel more relaxed immediately. And look a lot better too!

"Eighty percent of success is showing up."
Woody Allen

27

Add to Your Joy List

C.W. Metcalf learned the value of a "joy list" from a boy dying of cancer.

What do you put on such a list? *Anything that gives you joy now or has in the past.* Be very specific:

- Plunging into a cool shower after mowing the grass

- Feeling how effortlessly your whittling knife glides through a block of birch

- Listening to the songs your child makes up to entertain herself

- Seeing the welcoming smiles of your fellow volunteers on a community project

Try to add to your list several times a week, as you experience fresh joy or remember something from another time and place. When things get negative, pull out your list and read. The sense of joy will return.

"People who don't have nightmares don't have dreams." Robert Paul Smith

28

Candy Is Dandy

Chocolate has the same chemicals—endorphins—that wash over your brain when you're in love. If you feel like nobody cares and nobody is around to hug you and make it better, try a chocolate "kiss" on your sore ego or emotions.

Some companies have a cupboard stocked with chocolate for employees to use when the going gets rough. Wouldn't it be nice if that became a benefit everywhere?

"Don't be afraid to go out on a limb. That's where the fruit is." Arthur F. Lenehan

29

Silent Scream

When negative feelings build, letting it all out in a scream can be therapeutic. But not all settings are suitable for a full-throated, jungle-piercing Tarzan yell. Try screaming without sound. That's right, close your eyes, open your mouth as wide as you can, and imagine turning loose a blood-curdling, window-shattering scream.

It releases stress and looks ridiculous besides, a bonus for your stressed-out office mates.

"The crisis of yesterday is the joke of tomorrow." H. G. Wells

30

What's So Funny About This?

A man was listening to C.W. Metcalf's *Lighten Up* audiocassettes, a series that teaches how to look at life's lighter side. He wanted to finish the last tape and turned off the car while he did so. Finished, he thought, "I need to lock the car so nobody steals these tapes." After carefully locking and slamming the car door, he saw his car keys dangling from the ignition. Furious, he stormed off to call a locksmith. Ninety minutes and forty dollars later, the thought struck him: "This is ironic. I'm furious because of listening to these tapes about how to look at life's lighter side. Why don't I do what the tapes suggest?" He began to belly-laugh about what happened and determined he would use the story to illustrate the power of humor.

Find something funny, ridiculous, ironic, or silly about the painful situation you're in. Comedians help us do this all the time. Seeing the humor in a painful situation *while it's happening* is tougher, but yields even greater benefits.

> "The difficult we do immediately; the impossible takes a little longer." Slogan of the U.S. Army

31

Reframe It

An optimist says the glass of water is half full. The pessimist says it's half empty. The negativist says, "I'd rather have coffee." The basic facts are exactly the same—it's all how you look at it.

Psychologists call this "reframing." You can put a new frame around the events or people that are getting you down and come up with a different outlook. You can say "Rainy days are dreary," or you can reframe the situation and say, "I like rainy days because of the splashing, pattering sounds on the roof. I especially like to sleep in a room where I can hear the rain on the roof."

The classic reframing came from philosopher Friedrich Nietzsche: "Whatever doesn't kill me makes me stronger."

"Problems are only opportunities in work clothes." Henry J. Kaiser

32

Early to Bed

Do you snap at people more when you're tired? Are you more patient with irritating situations when you're not exhausted? Go to bed. A lot of things will look different and brighter in the morning.

Whatever you do to take care of your body and promote your good health will also help you manage your own and other people's negativity. Get plenty of rest, watch what you eat, breathe deeply, get in better cardiovascular and physical shape— you'll handle stress better and your body will thank you.

"The best way to make your dreams come true is to wake up." Paul Valery

33

Take a Deep Breath

Under stress, most people take shallow breaths. But this creates deficit spending in your breathing—you can keep going for a while, but eventually you may have to gasp to catch up again.

To handle stress better, consciously do the opposite. You have many more oxygen-handling receptors at the *bottom* of your lungs than at the top. Deeper breathing results in *significantly* more oxygen, and with that comes better physical and mental functioning.

Start by sitting up straight but comfortably. Let your head drop slightly forward as you close your eyes and let them turn downward to relax. Let your jaw relax as you focus on lengthening the time you take to exhale. Then lengthen the time it takes you to inhale until you are breathing in and breathing out very, very slowly.

In less than five minutes, you will be much calmer and more collected.

"Each handicap is like a hurdle in a steeplechase, and when you ride up to it, if you throw your heart over, the horse will go along too." Lawrence Bixby

Toys Aren't Just for Kids

People of all ages can get through tough times and stressful days by spending a few moments with a toy.

Visit the novelty shop and pick up a slinky, a screaming hatchet, a stress doll with removable limbs and head, a miniature basketball and wastebasket goal, some jacks, playdough, or whatever. When the tension mounts, take a break to play.

One company encourages its employees to help put together ongoing jigsaw puzzles. Anyone can place a piece or two as he or she walks by. Finished puzzles are glued, framed, and hung for all to admire and enjoy.

Try this at home too—to add some play time to the drudgery of housework or doing your taxes, or as "time out" during an argument with your teenager.

> "The secret of genius is to carry the spirit of the child into old age, which means never losing your enthusiasm." Aldous Huxley

35

Affirm It

The reticular formation of your brain determines what you will pay attention to in your conscious mind. You'd come unhinged if you tried to process on a conscious level everything your five senses are taking in. For instance, you generally aren't aware of your big toe unless it's too hot, too cold, stepped on, pinched by your shoe, or stung by a bee. Or you just read about toes.

As a hedge against negativity, you can tell your brain what you *choose* to have it focus on. It's a bit like goal setting carried one step higher.

Here's how a model affirmation comes together:

- State an emotion you'd feel if you reached your goal: *"I am confidently and joyfully ..."*

- State an action verb: *"... earning and investing ..."*

- Be specific about what you want: *"... $150,000 a year."*

Say the affirmation morning and night, and one of two things will happen: You'll keep using the affirmation, and it will help you subconsciously do the necessary things to reach your goal. Or you'll stop using the affirmation because you've changed goals or found another way to bolster your efforts.

"The best thing about the future is that it comes one day at a time." Anonymous

36

Rx: See Your Doctor

If your negativity is chronic, it *might* signal a health problem. Sometimes there's a physical explanation for being down emotionally.

A thyroid imbalance, for example—too much or too little—can definitely affect your moods. So can premenstrual swings in hormone levels. Are you taking an anti-inflammatory medication like prednisone for joint or bowel troubles? If so, this can make you feel edgy or easily angered.

Aside from ruling out causes such as these, don't overlook depression. Not the fleeting, "I'm depressed because I have to work this weekend" variety, but the persistent, ongoing kind that can rob you of energy (physical and emotional) and sap your sense of hope.

Seeing your doctor is the most positive prescription for dealing with the physical side of negativity.

> "One's attitude toward oneself is the single most important factor in healing and staying well." Bernie Siegel

37

Make It Worse

Fan the flames of your imagination ... how bad *could* things get? Pretend the worst scenario actually happened—what then?

For example, if you're concerned about losing your job due to "right-sizing," what's the worst outcome you can dream up? Losing your house? Going bankrupt? Suffering a family breakup?

As soon as we say out loud what *could* happen, we immediately start telling ourselves we would still survive. We start to plan how we'd make it ("I'd move in with my parents"). Sometimes our fears are just; at other times, because we're used to thinking negatively, they're only:

False

Evidence

Appearing

Real

> "The enemy is in front of us, behind us, to the left of us, and to the right of us. They can't escape us this time!" Marine Lieutenant Lewis B. (Chesty) Puller

38

Dial-a-Smile

Call someone who makes you feel good—your best buddy, a funny relative, a customer who always makes you feel like a million dollars.

How about contacting your favorite high school teacher? Tell that person how he or she made a difference in your life. You'll brighten both your days.

"Trouble is part of your life, and if you don't share it, you don't give the person who loves you a chance to love you enough." Dinah Shore

39

It's Contagious

You've heard since you were a kid that "birds of a feather flock together." But when it comes to the company you keep, remember the other old adage that goes "He that lieth down with dogs, riseth with fleas."

If you hang around negative people long enough, it's likely you'll become more negative yourself. Stay out of the cafeterias or breakroom if all you encounter are gripe sessions. Find positive, upbeat people to spend time with. Perhaps you can create an optimistic group, a "personal" board of directors to advise and encourage you when you're facing tough times or choices.

"The Wright brothers flew right through the smokescreen of impossibility." Charles F. Kettering

40

Use Your Mental Earplugs

Sometimes you'd probably like to plug your ears around someone who's demonstrating negative behavior, but you can't usually do that. However, you *can* insert "mental" earplugs.

The process is simple. Can you ignore negative remarks and *act as if* you didn't hear them? Is the person just blowing off steam? If so, it's wiser to say nothing.

Learn to distinguish between remarks you need to respond to and those you can ignore or tune out— those said in a heated moment, or those muttered by a someone who's demonstrated unwillingness to solve problems in the past.

"Some people are always grumbling because roses have thorns. I am thankful that thorns have roses." Alphonse Karr

41

Do the Can-Can

A young student of tae kwon do was having trouble breaking a board using a knife hand. The master came over and knelt in front of the child so they were eye to eye. He said, "Say, 'Yes, I can.'" The child responded, "Yes, I can." The master had the child say it three times, each time louder. Then he held the board up and said, "Break!" The student broke the board.

When faced with a major challenge, consider what you can do, not what you can't. Always spend more time *solving* problems than *talking* and *complaining* about them.

Say to the perpetual alarmist, "Thank you for raising that concern. Now what can we do to solve that or avoid that?" Especially if that alarmist is your own inner voice.

Just *thinking* you can helps makes the impossible possible. If you think you can't, you can't.

> "Those who dare do; those who dare not, do not." Anonymous

42

Ask the Right Questions

Anthony Robbins teaches the value of asking positively framed questions in his book titled *Awakening the Giant Within.* We are constantly asking ourselves questions, and if we're not careful, a lot of them will be negative: "What do I hate about my job?" "What's wrong with me?" "Why do we keep doing it this way?"

Learn to cast your questions positively—"What do I like about my job?" "What have I learned from this difficult situation?" "What's going well now?" "How can I improve this?"

One man turned a negative workplace around by repeatedly asking, "What did we do *right?*" First he was a solitary voice crying in a parched wilderness. Soon others were echoing his question to each other.

You and others will look at life differently when you ask the right questions.

"And what is a weed? A plant whose virtues have not been discovered." Ralph Waldo Emerson

43

Get Spiritual

Negativity comes when we feel out of control, helpless, without hope that anything we do matters. Many find their spiritual beliefs give new hope and a positive, long-term perspective.

Does your faith in a higher power cast your current situation in a better light? Let your current challenges take on a different look by viewing them with an eye turned toward eternity.

"Your mind is a sacred enclosure into which nothing harmful can enter except by your permission."
Arnold Bennet

44

Say "Ouch"

What was the worst physical pain you ever suffered? What about the worst emotional blow you or someone you know experienced? *This* isn't as bad as *that*, is it? If you can say "no," you will realize that things could be a lot worse!

If you survived that person, boss, place, or situation, you can and will survive this one!

"We acquire the strength we have overcome." Ralph Waldo Emerson

45

Up Your Stroke/Poke Ratio

You are your own coach, plus you also coach associates, friends, and family. Good coaches know when the player or team needs a figurative kick in the pants, but *great* coaches master the art of constant praise and encouragement, especially after a hard-fought defeat.

Experts say unless the strokes we get outnumber the pokes by at least four to one, we will perceive that the person giving the feedback views us in a negative way.

What is your stroke/poke ratio when you talk to others? What about when you talk to yourself? How often do you say something nice compared to how often you threaten or criticize?

If your stroke/poke ratio is less than four to one, make a conscious effort to up the strokes and limit the pokes. And treat yourself to the praise you'd like others to give you. Be the kind of coach you'd like to play for.

> "Luck is what happens when preparation meets opportunity." Darrell Royal

46

Hang It Up

Does your work space or home give you a boost? If not, post slogans, bumper stickers, plaques, signs, or cartoons that brighten your day and give you hope.

A successful corporate trainer keeps a handmade sign next to his overhead projector that reads, "Fast pace with enthusiasm." Every time the sign catches his eye, you can hear more energy in his voice. And you can see and hear it in his audience too.

"If you believe, and if you persist, all things are possible." Rieva Lesonsky

47

Don't Should on Yourself or Others

"Should" is a shame-based word for most of us. It comes from the same root as "scold." All that's missing is someone shaking an index finger at us while saying, "Shame, shame, shame!"

Use words that imply choice instead: "I *want* to." "I *get* to." "I *choose* to." "I *will!*" And if you catch yourself using "should," deliberately back up and substitute one of these other words that reaffirm your power to choose.

"Discontent is the first necessity of progress. Show me a thoroughly satisfied man and I will show you a failure." Thomas Alva Edison

48

Ain't It a Shame!

Guilt is feeling bad about what you *did*. *Shame* is feeling bad about what you *are*, about what an act says you're really like.

Guilt is hard enough to get over, but shame can be nearly impossible. How do you get rid of it? Find people you trust. People who will look you in the eye and not turn away. People who will speak to you with compassion, not condemnation. And in the right setting—people who can give you *safe* touch— a pat on the back, a touch on the elbow, or sometimes even a hug.

When someone hears what you are and still accepts you, your feelings of shame begin to fade. No wonder support groups and good counselors are so helpful! They give us a safe place to air our shame and release its power over us.

"I guess this means they fired me. I'll never make the mistake of being 70 years old again." Casey Stengel

49

Be Agreeable

Control freaks love to hear you say, "You're *right*."
They also like to hear the word *respect*. Can you find
something—anything—to agree about with a
disagreeable person?

How about, "You're *right*, we don't agree at all. But
I *respect* your *right* to look at it differently." Or how
about, "You're *right*, I don't understand what you
mean."

"The greatest pleasure in life is doing what
people say you cannot do." Walter
Bagehot

50

Trace Your Roots

Does someone on your family tree inspire you? Do you know stories about hardships they endured? You're from the same stock. You've got the same genetic "fuel" they had. If your relative did it, so can you!

Now look at your own personal history. Where did you start out? What obstacles have you already overcome? If you got through those challenges, you'll get through this one!

"If you can dream it, you can do it. Always remember that this whole thing was started by a mouse." Walt Disney

51

Change Your Hat

Will a change of mental headgear change your perspective? How about trading your "manager's hat" for your "friend," "co-worker," or "fellow human" hat?

Does this different hat help you see that difficult person or situation in a new light? Perhaps even with an improved, more positive perspective?

"Even if you're on the right track, you'll get run over if you just sit there." Will Rogers

52

Eyes on the Prize

When your present or past isn't so swift, shift your focus to the future. Is there a big event coming soon? Think how happy you'll be. Picture who'll be with you. What will you be doing? Where will you be? What will you wear?

Even little "big events" can get you through rough spots. Tell yourself, "It's only ___ days until Friday," or "It's only ____ weeks until my vacation."

Don't borrow troubles from the past, but *do* borrow joy from the future.

"Action is the antidote to despair." Joan Baez

53

Sounding Boards

When the noise of negativity is rattling your thoughts, seek a good listener, someone you trust, to be your sounding board. Ask him or her to refrain from trying to "fix things" or to solve your problem, but just to let you put what's bothering you into words. Ask your sounding board to repeat back what you've said.

Saying something aloud often helps you understand it better and see remedies you've been missing as you churned along.

"To be a real champion, you must believe you are the best. If you're not, pretend you are." Muhammad Ali

54

This Is Dedicated to the One I Love

Whom are you doing this for? You're willing to put up with a lot for (him, her, them), aren't you? He, she, or they are worth every bit of effort, right? Take a good long look at the person's picture. Glance at one of your love letters.

Dedicate this moment—and your willingness to endure whatever you're facing—to the one you love.

"The best way to cheer yourself up is to cheer everybody else up." Mark Twain

55

Put a Price Tag on It

Sure, this current situation may be rough. But are you getting paid for it?

Disney tells employees to remember that when they don't feel like smiling, they get *paid* to smile. When you're going through agony on the job, tell yourself, "Well, I'm getting paid $____ an hour (or a month) to put up with this."

"We will either find a way, or we will make one." Hannibal, about to cross the Alps with *elephants*

56

Shifting Gears

If you're upset about things at work, change the topic and think about things at home. If you're upset about things at home, think about work.

If both areas are troubling you, give your brain something else to think about. Noodle around with a puzzle. Read a book you've been wanting to pick up for months. Think of these diversions as short vacations for mental R&R. When your mind is refreshed, you can tackle your tough situation with renewed vigor.

"The things which hurt, instruct." Benjamin Franklin

57

3:2:1

An effective way to help yourself (or those you lead) to become more positive about change is called "3:2:1."

Ask everyone to list three things they liked about the old way of doing things, two things they didn't like, and one thing they thought could have been improved. Then ask for three things they like about the new way, two things they don't like, and one thing they think can be improved.

Negativity often comes out of vague, unarticulated fears or frustrations. By putting a "face" on each side of a challenge, you help those involved to become more *specific*, and thus more *positive*.

"The only way to avoid criticism is to do nothing, say nothing, be nothing." Elbert Hubbard

58

Step by Step

Many people enjoy running errands—the more, the better. They enjoy the sense of getting something done, of closure, of being able to cross things off their "to do" list.

Completing some minor "incompletes" frees up energy for you to deal with the bigger challenges that await your attention. If something's broken, fix it, sell it, or give it away. If it's out of style or doesn't fit and you don't wear it—pitch it, have a yard sale, or give it to charity.

Uncluttering your physical world unclutters your mental world too.

"Yesterday is a canceled check, tomorrow is a promissory note. Today is ready cash ... Use it!" Anonymous

59

Tape Your Negativity Shut

Even at your lowest ebb, you have access to a host of experts who stand ready to help you look at things differently and more positively.

Build your self-esteem with Jack Canfield. Tap into the power to act through Anthony Robbins. Find out the secrets of effective people from Stephen Covey. Look at life's lighter side with C.W. Metcalf.

If you could invite any of these people to ride in your car for an hour, what would it be worth to you? Wouldn't you jump at the chance? You *can* have them speak to you—on your car's audiocassette. And did you know you have the equivalent of two months' work time in your car to listen to these experts each year?

When you're down, nothing can help you get up more quickly than a motivational speaker at his or her best. And what's even better, a cassette player can go with you anywhere, and allow you to do two things at once. Walk and grow; commute and grow; clean house or work in the garden and grow. Leverage your attitude while you leverage your time.

"If you don't change your beliefs, your life will be like this forever. Is that good news?"
Robert Anthony

60

Try a Little Tenderness

Though you may find it easy (and quite natural) to pamper a friend going through hard times, do you extend the same sort of nurturing to yourself when you hit one of life's potholes? Emotional "chicken soup" sometimes works better and faster than all the pep talks you can muster. Do what you instinctively reach for …

Sleep late. Have a facial. Get a massage. Take a day off without an agenda. Skip your morning run. Indulge in several arrangements of fresh flowers. Have cheesecake for breakfast. Treat yourself to something special with the same energy and creativity that you'd expend on someone very dear to you. Because that's who you are.

> "The privilege of a lifetime is being who you are." Joseph Campbell

61

Under the Dumping Tree

Pick out a sturdy-looking tree a few blocks from home that you pass on the way to work. If you don't want to take personal problems to the office with you, mentally dump them off at the tree as you go by. Tell yourself they'll be there waiting when you come home.

You can also unload your work problems and worries at that maple or oak just before you turn onto your street. Pick them up again tomorrow after a good night's sleep and some R&R with your family.

"What the caterpillar calls the end of the world, the master calls a butterfly." Richard Bach

62

Extending a Helping Hand

People who volunteer their time seem to deal with significantly less negativity in their lives. Why? Because volunteers are people:

- Who have hope.

- Who are committed to *improving* things.

- Who get joy and satisfaction from helping others.

Volunteering has much to recommend it, not the least of which is how it helps avert your eyes from your own troubles. Part of your "paycheck" as a volunteer can be the graphic reminders of the blessings in your life.

And few things will register on your positivity meter like words of sincere thanks or a look of genuine appreciation from someone you've helped.

> "Only a life lived for others is the life worth living." Albert Einstein

63

Come to Your Senses

Spend a day concentrating on the sounds around you. Really hear them all. The sound of water gurgling down the drain. Then the sound of water splashing in the shower. Different, aren't they? Have you ever really heard them before?

Listen to your own footsteps in your slippers. In your shoes. On the oak hall floor. Now on the linoleum or the carpet.

What about a day devoted to sight? Colors. Shadows. The sun. Reflections. Shiny. Dull. Metallic. Fluorescent light. Incandescent light. Track lights. Tail lights. Candlelight. Transparent. Translucent.

Devote another day to feel and touch. Continue your journey on another day by really smelling your world—a bath towel right out of the dryer, freshly seasoned food, your perfume, your car, your office.

Do you feel more alive? More alert? Now what was it you were troubled about?

"What a wonderful life I've had. I only wish I had realized it sooner." Collette

64

Learn Something New

Students of all ages feel a surge of optimism at the onset of a new school year. That annual recommitment to personal growth and learning brings a jolt of positivity along with it. Though it's difficult sometimes to learn new things, there's a lot of "up" in rising to a challenge.

For instance, learn to use some new software that stretches your repertoire of skills. Take a class at your local junior college or technical school. What have you always been interested in but didn't have the time to pursue? Take the time now. Even a once-a-week class will energize you as you begin to feel the sleepy parts of your mind wake up. Learn to cook, draw, paint, write, work on your car—whatever you've dreamed of being able to do or know. You'll not only polish your golf swing or improve your French accent—the focusing will fine-tune your outlook as well.

> "Anyone who stops learning is old, whether at twenty or eighty." Henry Ford

65

Philosophy of Positivity

Forrest Gump put a positive spin on uncertainty by demonstrating how life is like a box of chocolates. Can you create a maxim or proverb to reflect how you look at life?

Here are some examples to get you started:

- "Good, bad, or indifferent, nothing lasts forever."

- "I'm breathing, my heart is pumping, and that sure beats the alternative!"

Maybe you can even get a T-shirt printed to spread your helpful philosophy: "I survived the audit of '96!"

"Believe that life is worth living and your belief will help create the fact." William James

66

Take Over the Controls

Examine the situations where you're feeling trapped or out of control. Do you have other options? When you look at all the consequences of the alternatives you have, you may still make the choice you originally thought you had to make. But now you will feel better, because you will know it's the action you chose to take. And that feels very different.

Viktor Frankl, psychologist and prisoner of war in Nazi Germany, said that between any stimulus and the response to it lies choice. Frankl decided his captors could limit his movements, diet, and activities, but they couldn't control his mind. They could limit his *liberties*, but they couldn't take away his *freedom*—that *he* controlled in his mind. He thus survived, and even thrived, in a hellish existence.

Taking control is crucial in eliminating negative thinking.

"While we may not be able to control all that happens to us, we can control what happens inside us." Ben Franklin

67

Testing 1 . . . 2 . . . 3

One way to overcome objections of the negativist is to say, "You may be right. But let's just test it for 30 days. Let's agree to give it our best shot for 30 days. We'll evaluate it in 30 days."

Not a bad personal strategy, either. If you've voiced your objections to new procedures and they still get implemented, try the same methodology. Tell yourself, "Well, I'm going to test this for 90 days. I'll give it 110 percent for three months. Then I'll sit down and see whether my concerns were valid."

After giving a fair effort to make the change work, you'll either be sold on the change or have better data to prove it isn't working.

"Ain't no chance if you don't take it." Guy Clark

68

Do Your Dirty Work

What's something you need to do that you've been putting off? Cleaning the garage? Organizing your closets or drawers? Painting the house? Sorting your files?

Do it! It'll give you a giant boost.

It's a boost, because the long-procrastinated project is finally off your mind. Sometimes we create more tension and fatigue *thinking* about getting something done than we would if we'd just do it.

"Things turn out best for people who make the best of the way things turn out." Art Linkletter

Back to the Future

Before you relinquish all sense of proportion, imagine you can "fast forward" the tape of your problem. How will it look in (take your pick):

> One year?

> Five years?

> A hundred years?

Shriveled? Dusty? Invisible? What seems so important today eventually loses its power. Though time perhaps can't heal *all* wounds, it does patch up most of them.

"God gave us a memory that we might have roses in December." James M. Barrie

70

Time Out

No, don't send yourself or your associate to the corner. But when tempers and nostrils flare, time to cool off may be just the prescription for healing.

When you're about to lose it, say: "I need a few minutes to think this over. I don't want to say something I'll regret." A step back will give you time to analyze the situation and choose carefully what you want to say.

When someone else is losing it with you, suggest: "I can tell you've got a lot to say. Why don't you take a minute or two to decide how you want to say it."

The few moments it takes to get a Coke or cup of coffee can douse out-of-control feelings and reestablish a sense of perspective.

> "If you are patient in one moment of anger, you will escape a hundred days of sorrow." Chinese proverb

71

Go, Team, Go!

Teams are changing America's workplace. Why? Because as Roy Disney put it, "None of us is as smart as all of us."

Could some of your problems be solved better by team input or a group approach? If you've rowed yourself off onto an island of worry, despair, and frustration, rejoin the human race! Looking at it another way, do you just let yourself suffer and stew when you don't know how to spell a word, or do you reach for the dictionary without embarrassment? Reaching out and tapping into the collective resources of a team is no different, and you'll find perspective as well as answers.

"Whatever the mind can conceive and believe, it can achieve." Napoleon Hill

72

Quitting Time

Quit. Really? Isn't that giving up? Isn't that reckless advice? No. Life is too short to spend 40 or 50 years of it being miserable.

Yes, do all you can to improve your situation or survive it. Yes, realize that in some way you are part of the problem. Yes, hope that things will get better. Yes, consider a lateral move or leave of absence if you work. No, don't burn your bridges. But at some point, be ready to get out and move on.

It hurts to lance a boil or to clean out a wound with peroxide. But healing won't happen until that pain is endured.

Saying "No more!" might just be the most positive words you'll ever speak.

> "A man who trims himself to suit everybody will soon whittle himself away." Charles M. Schwab

73

Climb to Common Ground

Too often when we focus on our differences, we highlight and underscore the negatives in our interactions.

How about turning the tables and first looking at where we *agree* on several key points? Discovering where we stand on common ground sends the positive message, "We're not as far apart as it first seemed!"

Once the group feels "shoulder to shoulder," list the areas of disagreement. Decide on which to talk about first. Agree to focus on that issue only until reaching a solution everyone can live with. Then move on to the next.

"I challenge you to double the amount of energy and enthusiasm you are putting into your life. I guarantee you will triple your feelings of self-esteem, happiness, and success." Connie Palladino

A Word From the Wise

In the words of an old proverb, "The way of a fool seems right to him, but a wise man listens to advice." Who could serve in this situation as your counselor, advisor, mentor? Seek that person out.

When a problem looks too big to tackle, take a moment to ask, "Who would best be able to advise me about this?"

Being smart isn't knowing all the answers. It's knowing when and where to find them.

"Success is not a destination, a place you can ever get to; it is the quality of your journey." Jennifer Jones

75

Do Nothing

Have you ever noticed how something that troubles you greatly one day may not seem so bad the next? One reason is that a good night's sleep or some time away from a problem can give you a clearer head and a new perspective. Plus some problems go away, resolve themselves, or get solved by others before you do a thing.

Don't ignore problems. But just as silence can be a powerful communication tool, a deliberate, planned period of inactivity can be a powerful strategy in dealing with sensitive or volatile issues. Letting some of the negativity dissipate or "boil off" can sometimes make a situation more receptive to solutions.

"The truly free man is he who knows how to decline a dinner invitation without giving an excuse." Jules Renard

76

Reward Yourself

When you've handled a negative situation, reward yourself. Decide what the reward will be before you take the tough steps, and don't fail to deliver.

Jack Canfield recommends setting aside a percentage of your income (1%) as a victory fund. You must use this money to do something for yourself you otherwise couldn't afford, or wouldn't "waste" money on. Take a limousine when you go out to dinner. Go skydiving. Get glamour photos made.

On a more modest scale, reward yourself with a reading break after you spend two hours cleaning the garage. Or with a pizza on Saturday after you eat sensibly all week.

Knowing a reward is coming can help you do the things you have to do but don't want to do. The carrot on a stick routine is not just for rabbits!

"Great works are performed not by strength but by perseverance." Samuel Johnson

77

Script It

Can you predict what you will fight about with your favorite "sparring" partner? Do you know your lines? Want to write a new play?

Jot down the dialog you've both used in the past over a familiar issue. Then examine your lines. Do they say what you'd like to say? Write a new part for yourself and rehearse with a "stand-in."

When you're comfortable saying your new lines, you're ready for a live performance. You'll find that when your lines change for the better, so will those of your antagonist.

"Never give in! Never give in! Never, never, never. Never—in anything great or small, large or petty—never give in except to convictions of honor and good sense."
Winston Churchill

78

Danger! Keep Out!!

You wouldn't wander into a burning building or pick up a rattler just because it happened to be in your path. Are you doing this to yourself in other parts of your life?

- Do you hang around people who put you down and pull the triggers to negative thoughts?

- Do you go to the grocery store hungry after successfully completing a long stretch of dieting?

- Does your mouth say "No problem!" when your head says "No way!"?

Don't just carefully identify the negative areas in your life. Try to see whether you can avoid or eliminate some of them by carefully planning one or two steps before the negativity sets in, and then adjusting your life accordingly.

> "Anybody can become angry—that is easy. But to be angry with the right person, to the right degree, at the right time, for the right reason, and in the right way—that is not easy." Aristotle

79

Whine Country

Here's what to do with a whine lover. Say, with a smile, "Would you like a little cheese?" When the nay-brayer looks puzzled or asks what you mean, say, "Would you like a little cheese to go with your whine?" Usually you will get a sheepish grin and the person's attitude will shift at least temporarily.

Humor can make target practice of negativity.

"You only live once, but if you work it right, once is enough." Joe E. Lewis

80

Rela-a-a-a-x

A relaxation exercise often gives a big shove to a bout of negativity.

Sit in a comfortable chair and rest your hands lightly on the arms of the chair. Lean your head back and roll your eyes upward and back as far as you can. Count slowly from ten to one, allowing your eyes to close slowly so that by the time you reach one, they are closed.

Now visualize yourself walking on a forest path. The wind in the trees overhead makes a soft swishing sound and moves the dappled sunlight around on the ground. The birds twitter and the squirrels chatter. As you leisurely stroll along the path, you can smell the tang of the ocean in the distance. You break out of the forest and stand on a cliff overlooking the sea. You spot a descending pathway and carefully begin to pick your way down. Seagulls scream and soar overhead. When you reach the beach, you are pleasantly tired and notice a stand of leafy bushes at the base of the cliff. You approach and lie down in the warm sun, shielding your face with the branches of the bushes. You close your eyes and begin to count the waves as they roll up on the shore. Each wave washes you deeper and deeper into relaxation. Begin to breathe in deeply with each wave that hits the shore and then breathe out as the wave slides along the sand back to the sea. Do this for as long as you are comfortable.

Open your eyes very slowly and feel how relaxed and refreshed you are.

"Stand tall. The difference between towering and cowering is totally a manner of inner posture. It's got nothing to do with height, it costs nothing, and it's more fun."
Malcolm Forbes

Bibliography and Suggested Reading

Braham, Barbara J. *Finding Your Purpose: A Guide to Personal Fulfillment.* Menlo Park, CA: Crisp Publications, 1989.

Canfield, Jack. *How to Build High Self-Esteem.* Chicago: Nightingale Conant, 1982.

Chapman, Elwood N. *Life Is an Attitude.* Los Altos, CA: Crisp Publications, 1991.

Cousins, Norman. *Anatomy of an Illness, As Perceived by the Patient: Reflections on Healing and Recognition.* Toronto: Bantam, 1981.

Covey, Stephen R. *The Seven Habits of Highly Effective People.* New York: Simon and Schuster, 1989.

Edelston, Martin, and Marion Buhagiar. *I-Power: The Secrets of Great Business in Bad Times.* Fort Lee, NJ: Barricade Books, 1992.

Hathaway, Patti. *Giving and Receiving Criticism: Practical Techniques for Interpersonal Effectiveness.* Los Altos, CA: Crisp Publications, 1990.

Metcalf, C. W. *Lighten Up! Survival Skills for People Under Pressure.* Niles, MI: Nightingale-Covenant, 1994.

Orstein, Robert E. *The Healing Brain: Breakthrough Discoveries About How the Brain Keeps Us Healthy.* New York: Simon and Schuster, 1987.

Palladino, Connie. *Developing Self-Esteem: A Positive Guide for Personal Success.* Los Altos, CA: Crisp, 1989.

Robbins, Anthony. *Awakening the Giant Within: How to Take Immediate Control of Your Mental, Emotional, Physical, and Financial Destiny.* New York: Summit Books, 1991.

Tracy, Brian. *The Phoenix Seminar.* Solano Beach, CA: Brian Tracy, 1990.

Available From SkillPath Publications

Self-Study Sourcebooks

Climbing the Corporate Ladder: What You Need to Know and Do to Be a Promotable Person *by Barbara Pachter and Marjorie Brody*

Coping With Supervisory Nightmares: 12 Common Nightmares of Leadership and What You Can Do About Them *by Michael and Deborah Singer Dobson*

Defeating Procrastination: 52 Fail-Safe Tips for Keeping Time on Your Side *by Marlene Caroselli, Ed.D.*

Discovering Your Purpose *by Ivy Haley*

Going for the Gold: Winning the Gold Medal for Financial Independence *by Lesley D. Bissett, CFP*

Having Something to Say When You Have to Say Something: The Art of Organizing Your Presentation *by Randy Horn*

The Innovative Secretary *by Marlene Caroselli, Ed.D.*

Mastering the Art of Communication: Your Keys to Developing a More Effective Personal Style *by Michelle Fairfield Poley*

Organized for Success! 95 Tips for Taking Control of Your Time, Your Space, and Your Life *by Nanci McGraw*

P.E.R.S.U.A.D.E.: Communication Strategies That Move People to Action *by Marlene Caroselli, Ed.D.*

Productivity Power: 250 Great Ideas for Being More Productive *by Jim Temme*

Promoting Yourself: 50 Ways to Increase Your Prestige, Power, and Paycheck *by Marlene Caroselli, Ed.D.*

Proof Positive: How to Find Errors Before They Embarrass You *by Karen L. Anderson*

Risk-Taking: 50 Ways to Turn Risks Into Rewards *by Marlene Caroselli, Ed.D. and David Harris*

Stress Control: How You Can Find Relief From Life's Daily Stress *by Steve Bell*

The Technical Writer's Guide *by Robert McGraw*

Total Quality Customer Service: How to Make It Your Way of Life *by Jim Temme*

Write It Right! A Guide for Clear and Correct Writing *by Richard Andersen and Helene Hinis*

Handbooks

The ABC's of Empowered Teams: Building Blocks for Success *by Mark Towers*

Assert Yourself! Developing Power-Packed Communication Skills to Make Your Points Clearly, Confidently, and Persuasively *by Lisa Contini*

Breaking the Ice: How to Improve Your On-the-Spot Communication Skills
by Deborah Shouse

The Care and Keeping of Customers: A Treasury of Facts, Tips, and Proven Techniques for Keeping Your Customers Coming BACK! *by Roy Lantz*

Challenging Change: Five Steps for Dealing With Change *by Holly DeForest and Mary Steinberg*

Dynamic Delegation: A Manager's Guide for Active Empowerment *by Mark Towers*

Every Woman's Guide to Career Success *by Denise M. Dudley*

Great Openings and Closings: 28 Ways to Launch and Land Your Presentations With Punch, Power, and Pizazz *by Mari Pat Varga*

Hiring and Firing: What Every Manager Needs to Know *by Marlene Caroselli, Ed.D. with Laura Wyeth, Ms.Ed.*

How to Be a More Effective Group Communicator: Finding Your Role and Boosting Your Confidence in Group Situations *by Deborah Shouse*

How to Deal With Difficult People *by Paul Friedman*

Learning to Laugh at Work: The Power of Humor in the Workplace *by Robert McGraw*

Making Your Mark: How to Develop a Personal Marketing Plan for Becoming More Visible and More Appreciated at Work *by Deborah Shouse*

Meetings That Work *by Marlene Caroselli, Ed.D.*

The Mentoring Advantage: How to Help Your Career Soar to New Heights *by Pam Grout*

Minding Your Business Manners: Etiquette Tips for Presenting Yourself Professionally in Every Business Situation *by Marjorie Brody and Barbara Pachter*

Misspeller's Guide *by Joel and Ruth Schroeder*

Motivation in the Workplace: How to Motivate Workers to Peak Performance and Productivity *by Barbara Fielder*

NameTags Plus: Games You Can Play When People Don't Know What to Say *by Deborah Shouse*

Networking: How to Creatively Tap Your People Resources *by Colleen Clarke*

New & Improved! 25 Ways to Be More Creative and More Effective *by Pam Grout*

The Power of Positivity: Eighty ways to energize your life *by Joel and Ruth Schroeder*

Power Write! A Practical Guide to Words That Work *by Helene Hinis*

Putting Anger to Work For You! *by Ruth and Joel Schroeder*

Reinventing Your Self: 28 Strategies for Coping With Change *by Mark Towers*

Saying "No" to Negativity: How to Manage Negativity in Yourself, Your Boss, and Your Co-Workers *by Zoie Kaye*

The Supervisor's Guide: The Everyday Guide to Coordinating People and Tasks *by Jerry Brown and Denise Dudley, Ph.D.*

Taking Charge: A Personal Guide to Managing Projects and Priorities *by Michal E. Feder*

Treasure Hunt: 10 Stepping Stones to a New and More Confident You! *by Pam Grout*

A Winning Attitude: How to Develop Your Most Important Asset! *by Michelle Fairfield Poley*

For more information, call 1-800-873-7545.